Lyme, One Day at a Time

Shannon Marie

My Mom hung up the phone
and called upstairs, "Come here please."

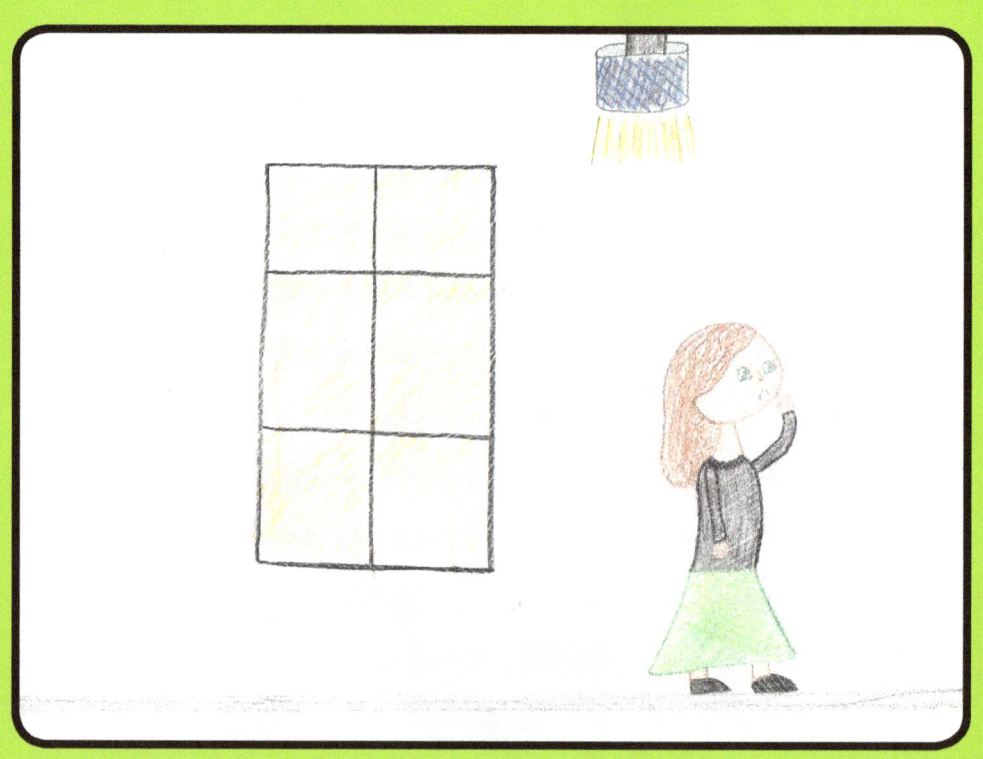

I sat down right beside her.

My dear one, you have Lyme disease.

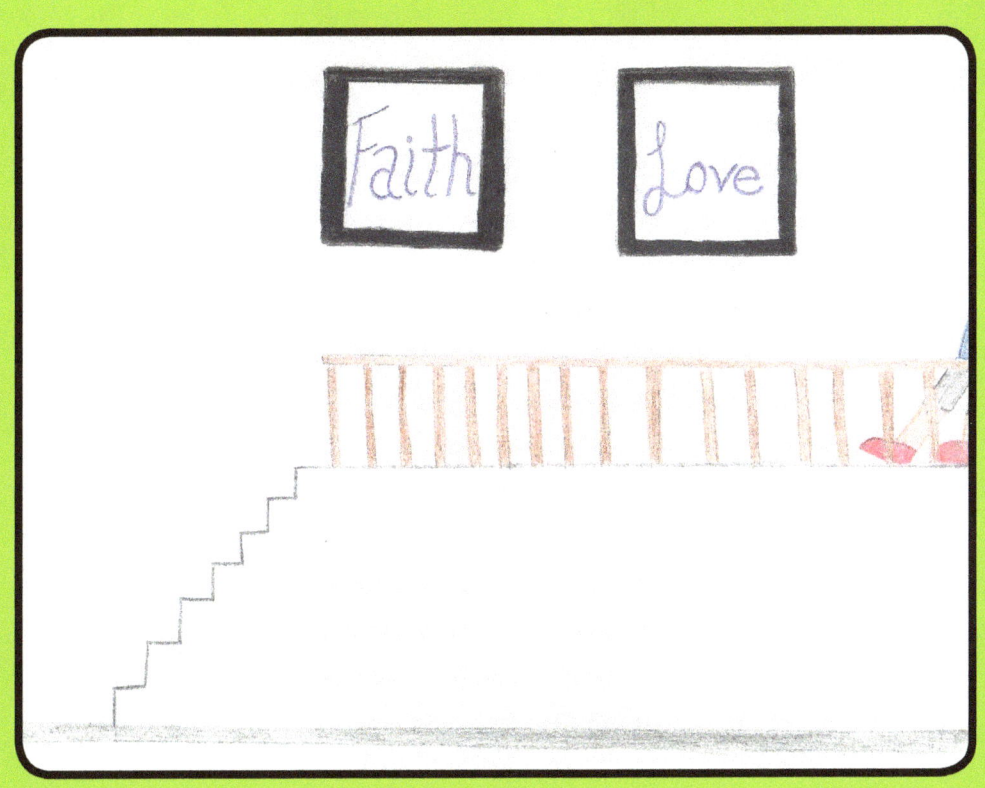

What is that? I pondered.

What is Lyme?

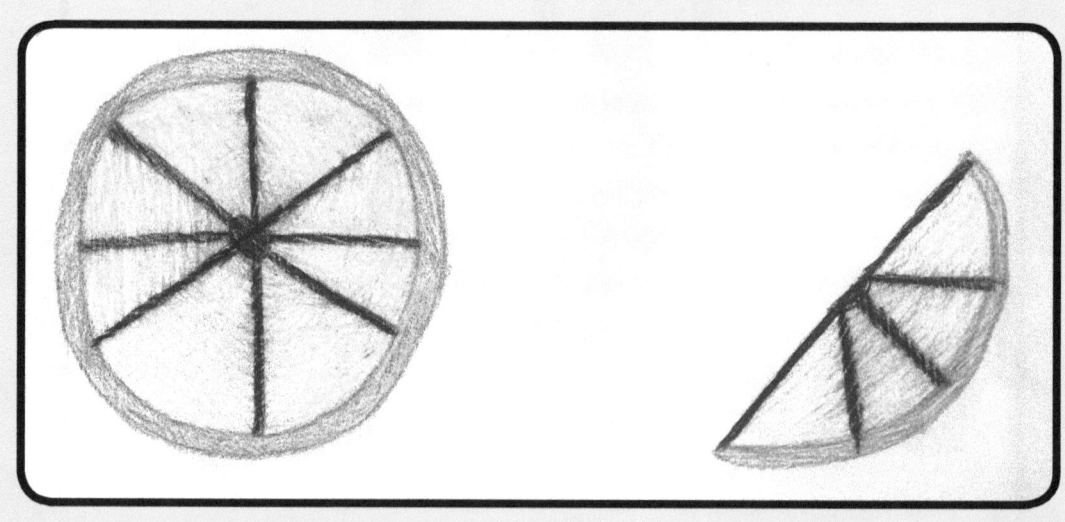

"Like the fruit Mom?"

No honey, Mom smiled, not lime. Lyme.

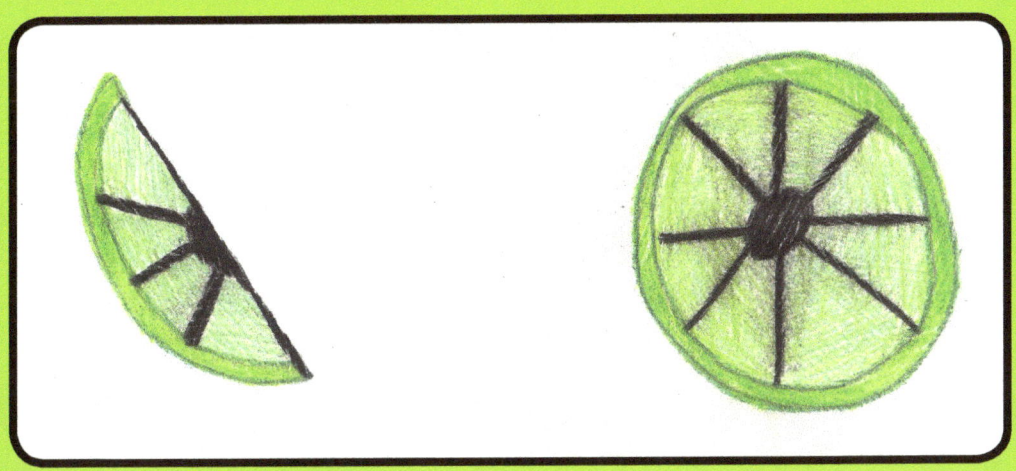

It can come from a tick,

a mite, mosquito or flea.

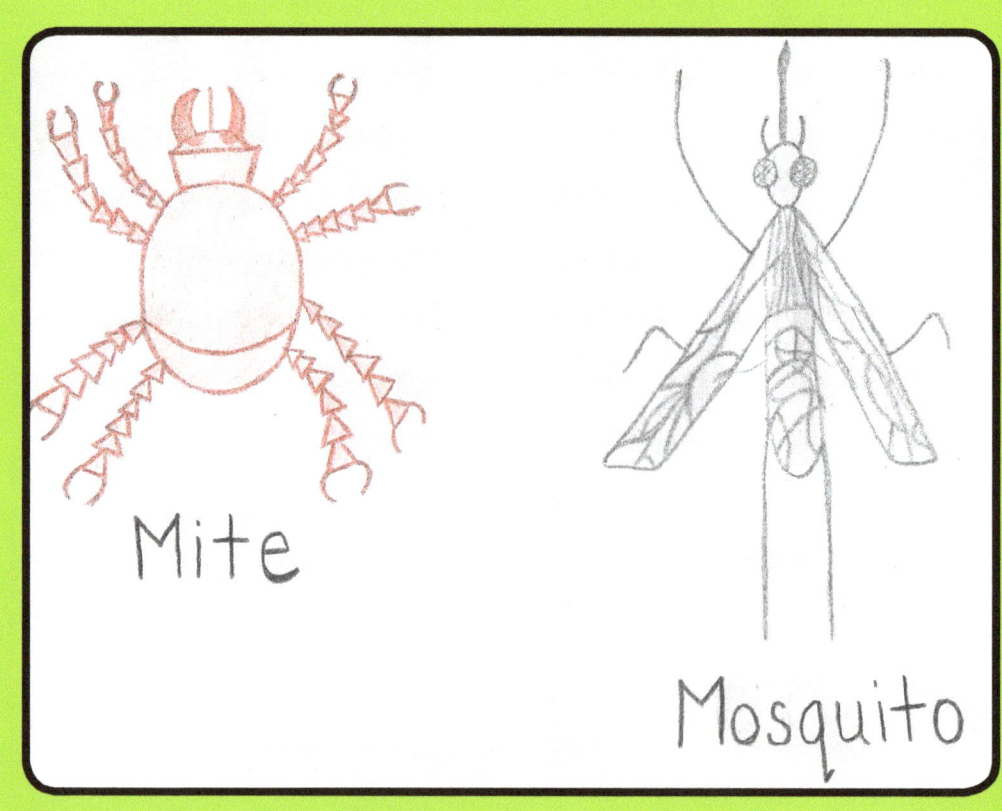

Mite

Mosquito

It can even be passed from
a Mother to her unborn baby.

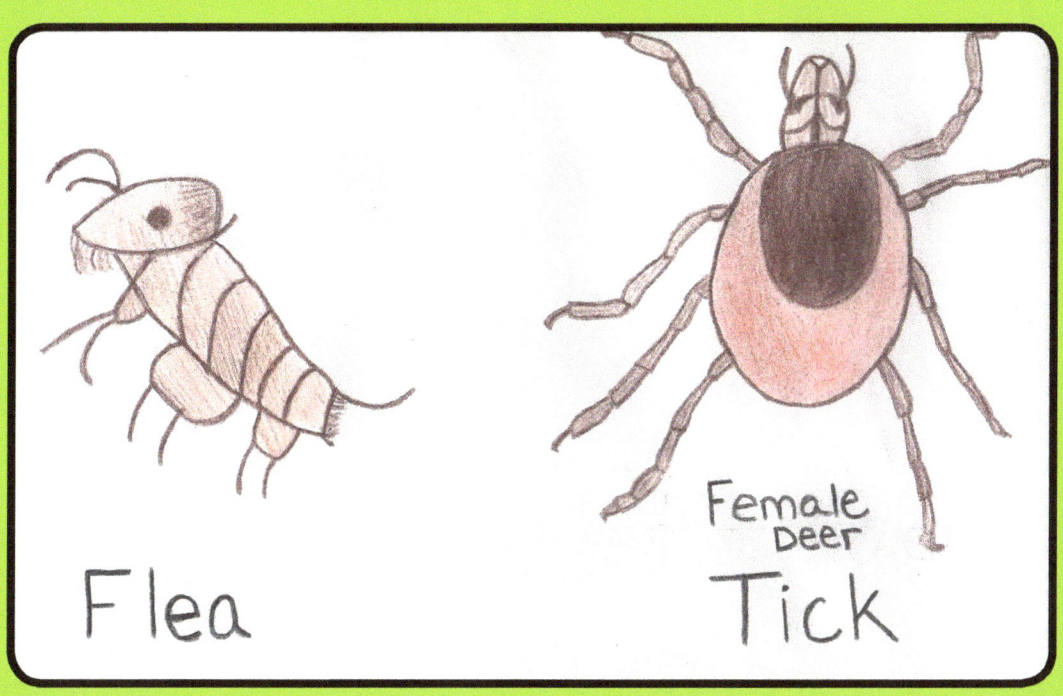

Flea

Female
Deer
Tick

The boy grew very sad.

He even began to cry.

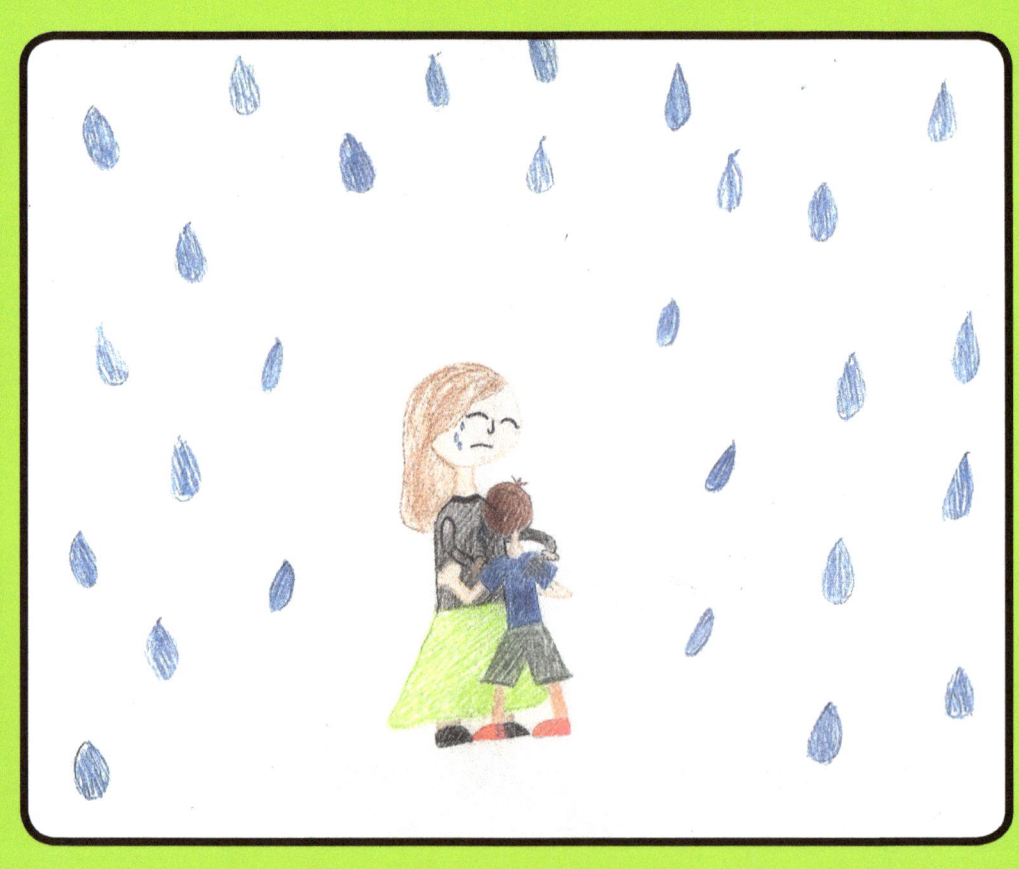

Mom, am I different from other kids?

Mom, am I going to die?

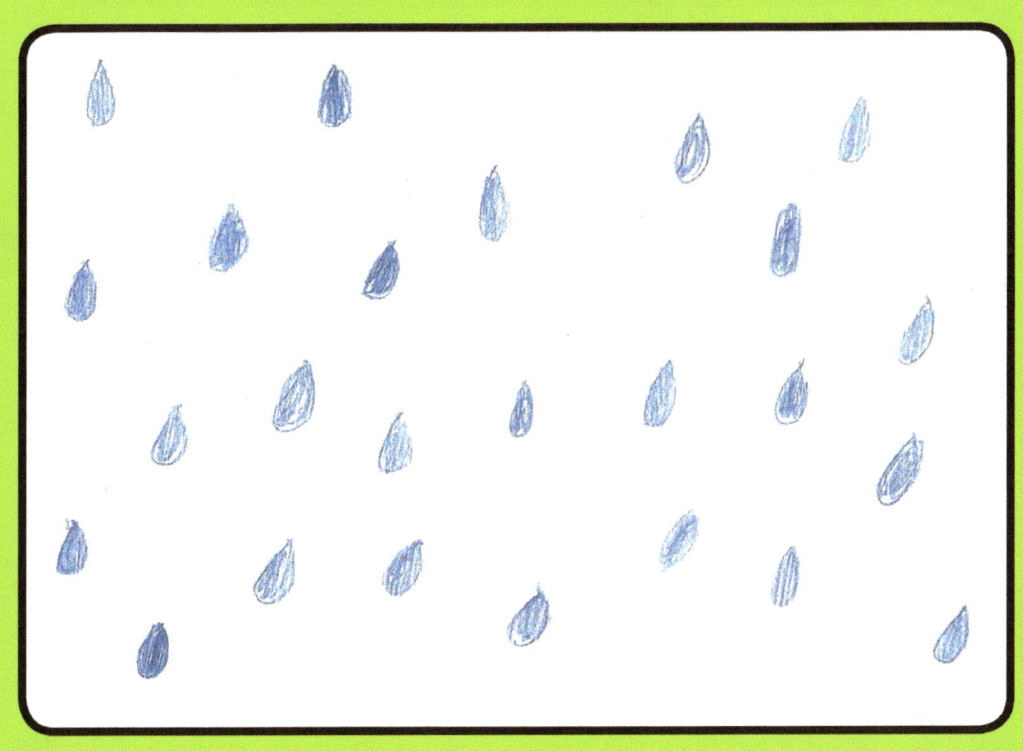

His Mom looked him in the eye
as she held him very tight.

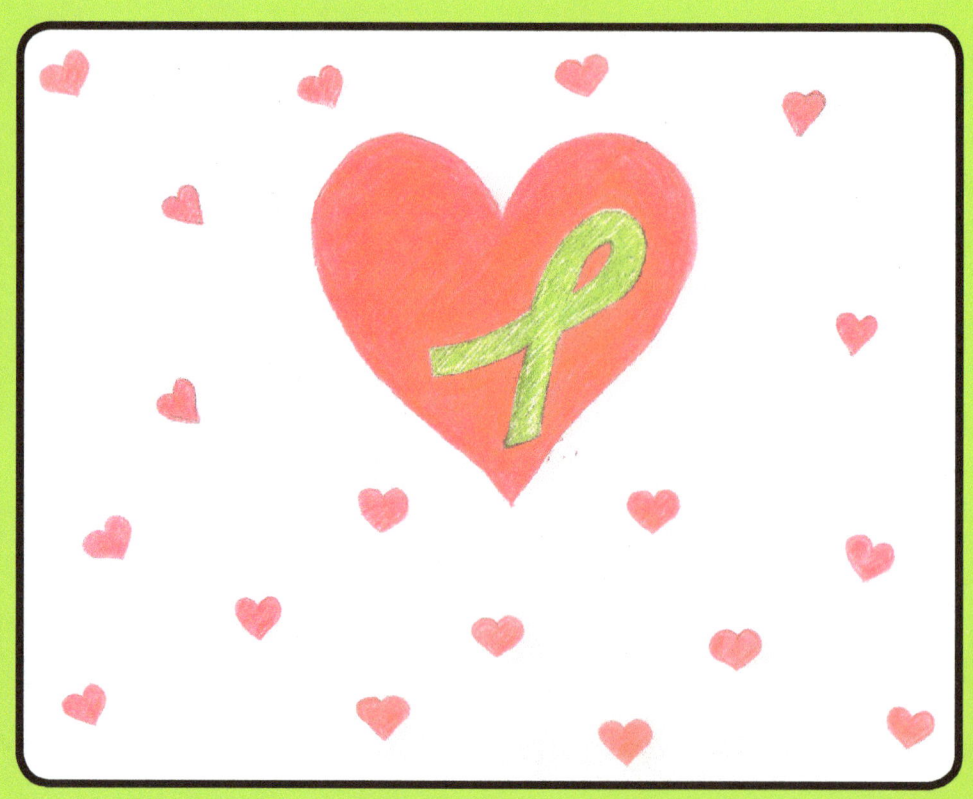

We will get through this together.

I love you; you're going to be alright.

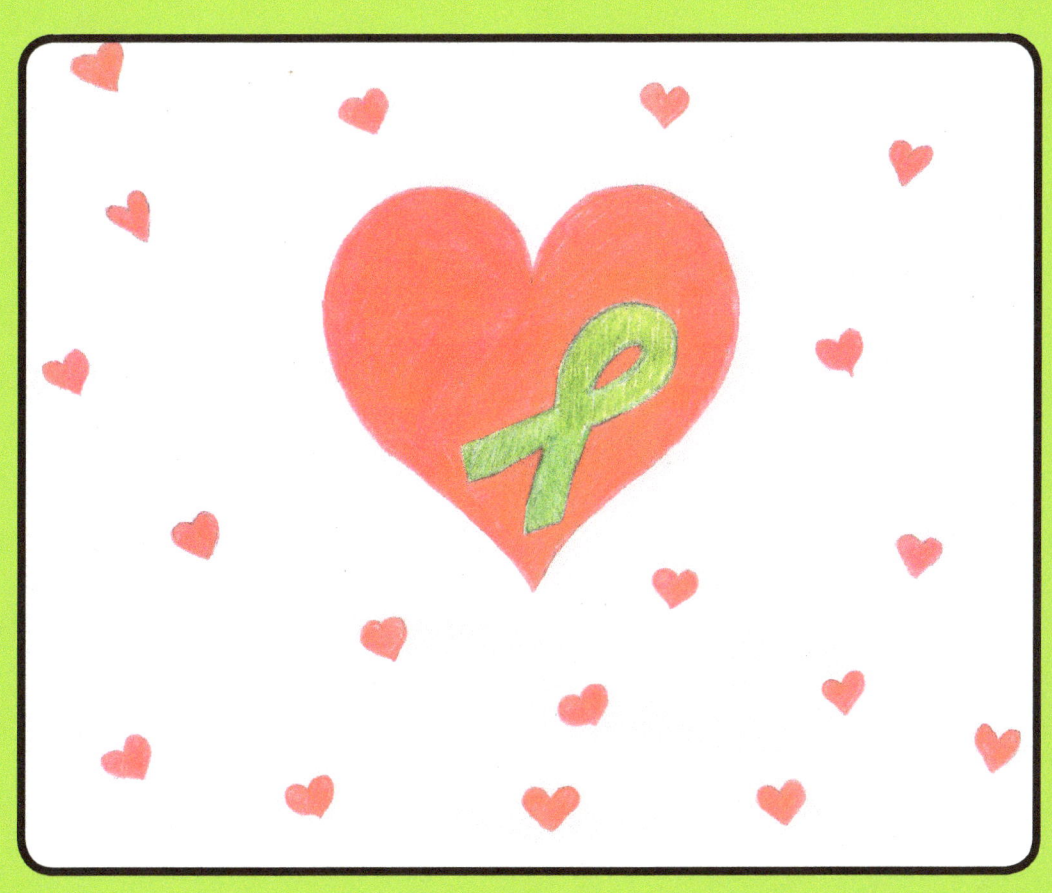

Don't look at this disease
as being different from the rest.

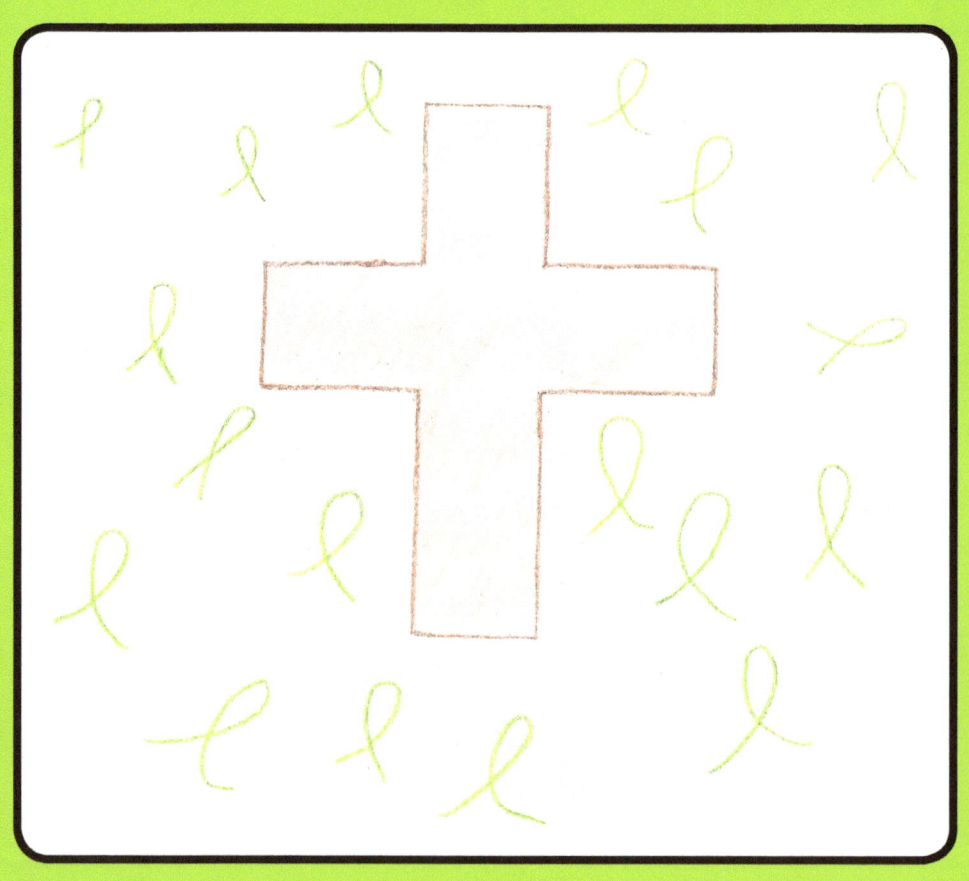

Look at it as opportunity

to trust in the very best!

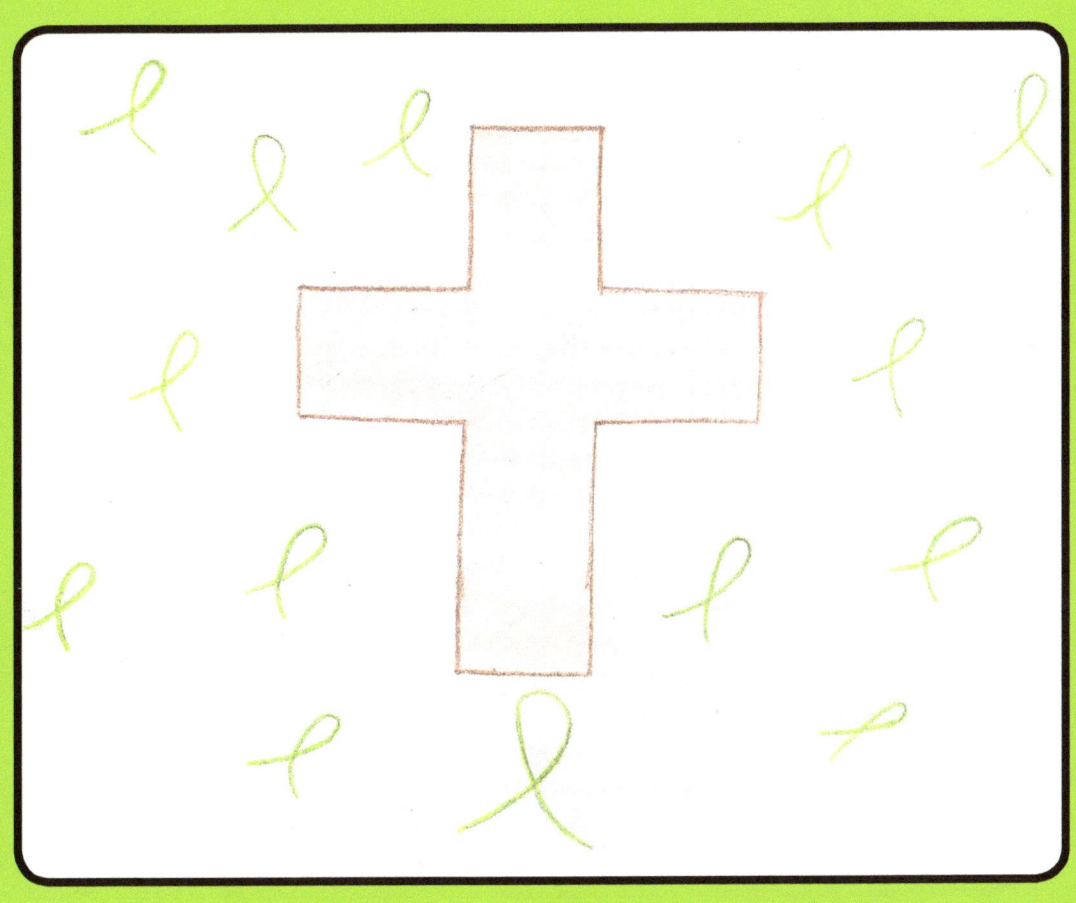

Yes, you will need to heal.

Yes, it can be a long ride.

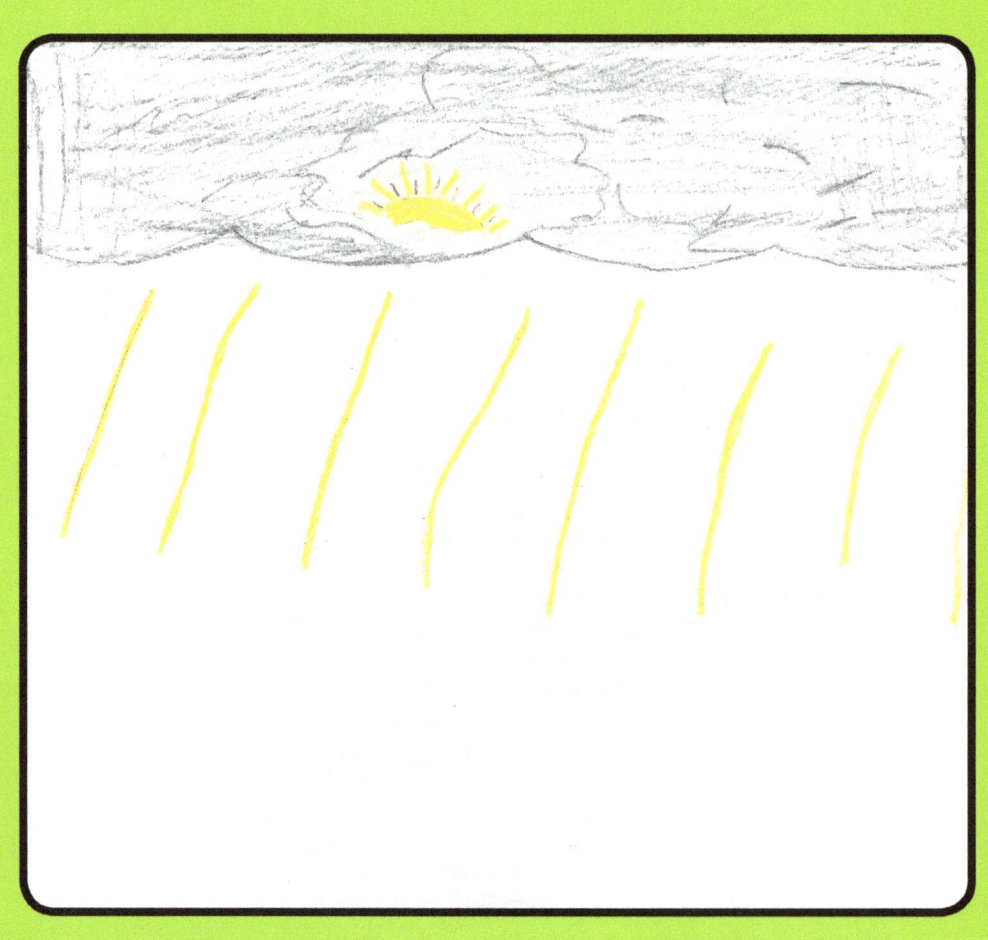

One day at a time, to remember,

the Lord is by your side.

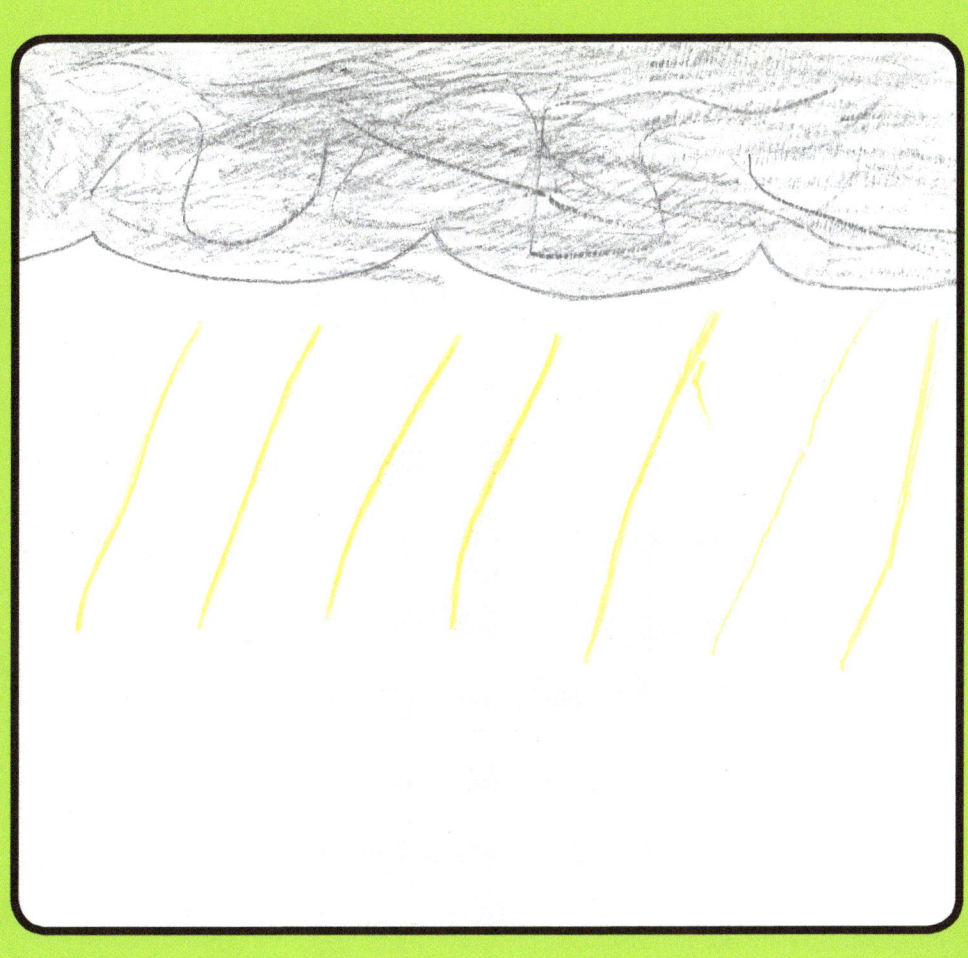

Don't focus on the battle son.

Focus on your Savior; your Superstar!

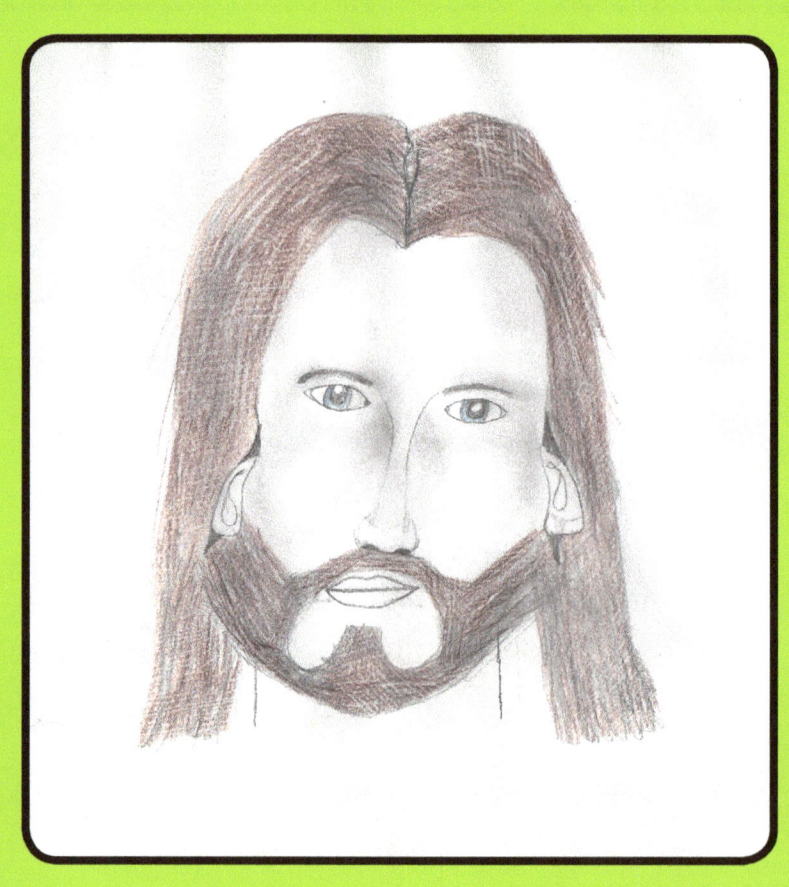

Lyme is just a disease.

It is NOT WHO YOU ARE!

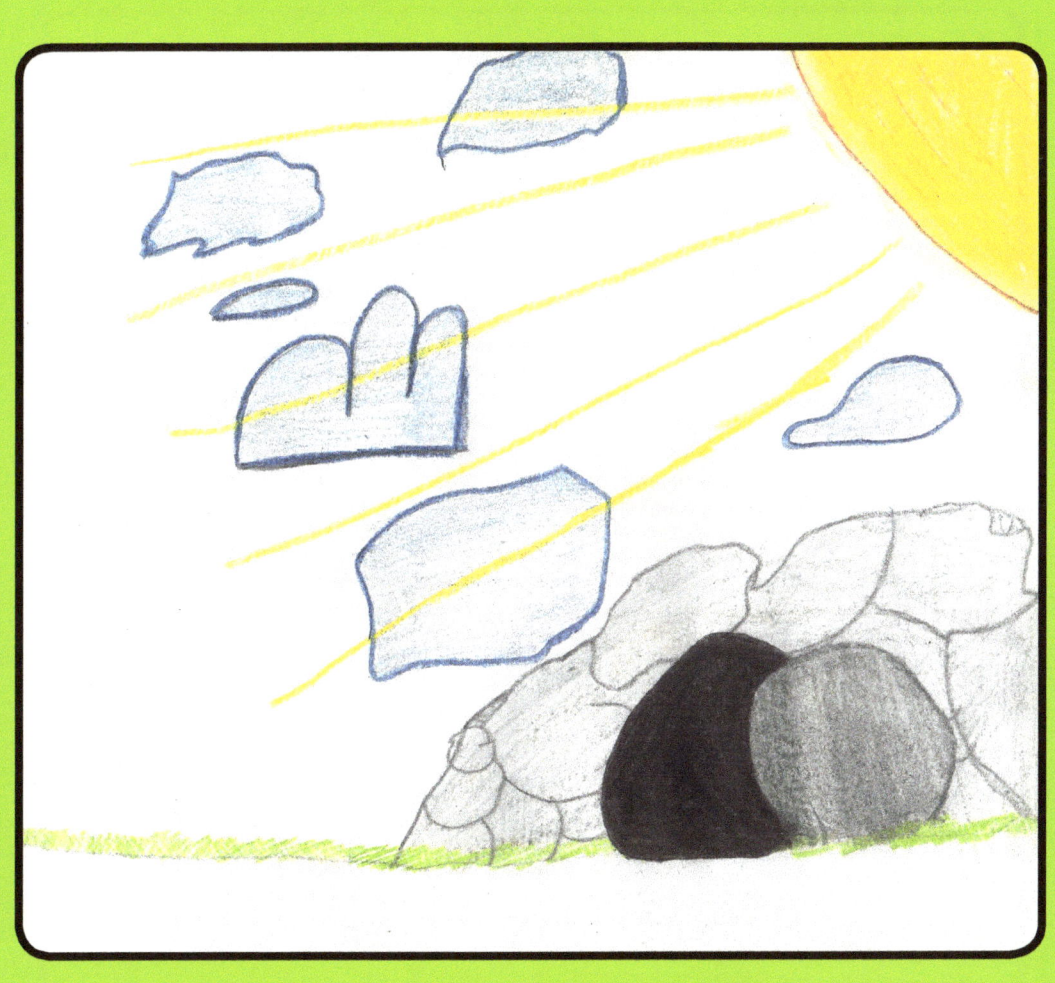

Okay Mom, I think I'm ready!

Let's win the battle ahead!

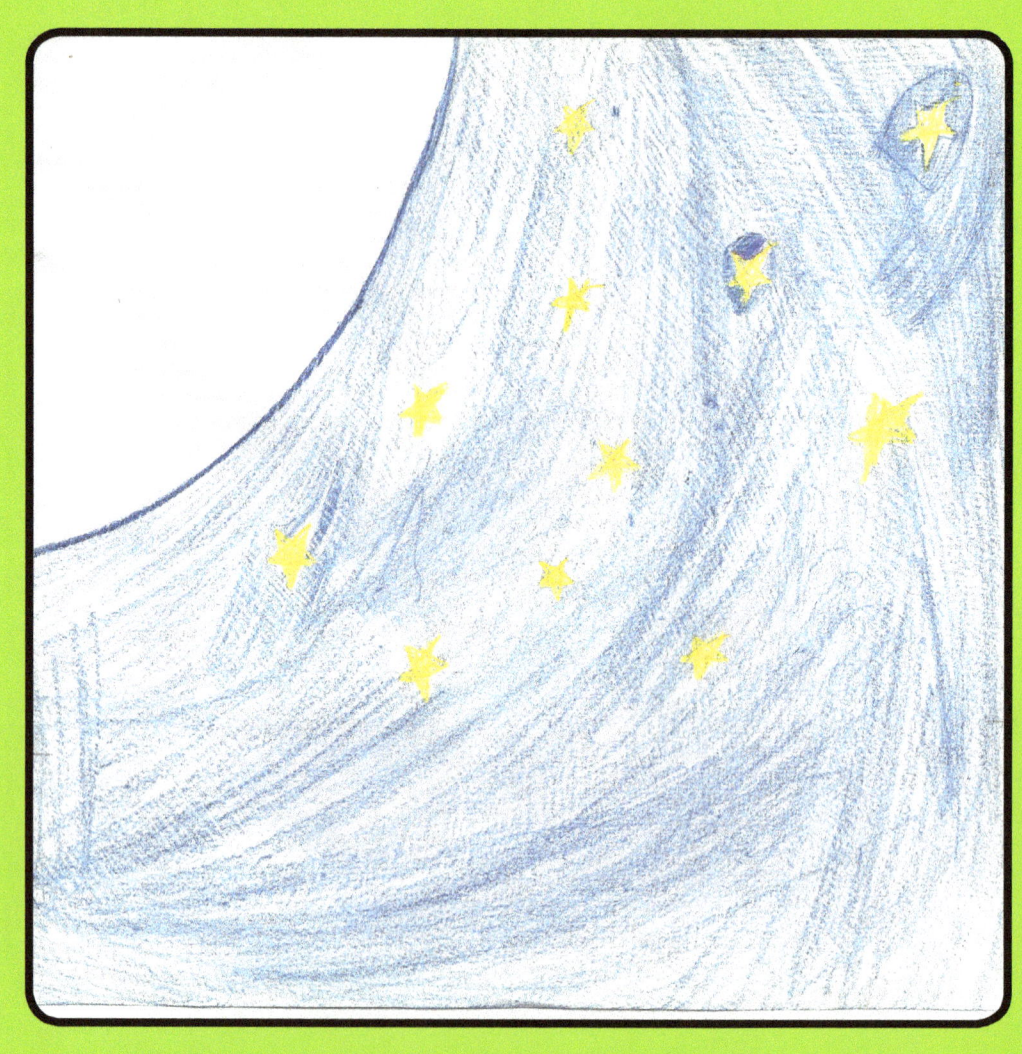

The Mom hugged her son;
let's pray and then it is time for bed.

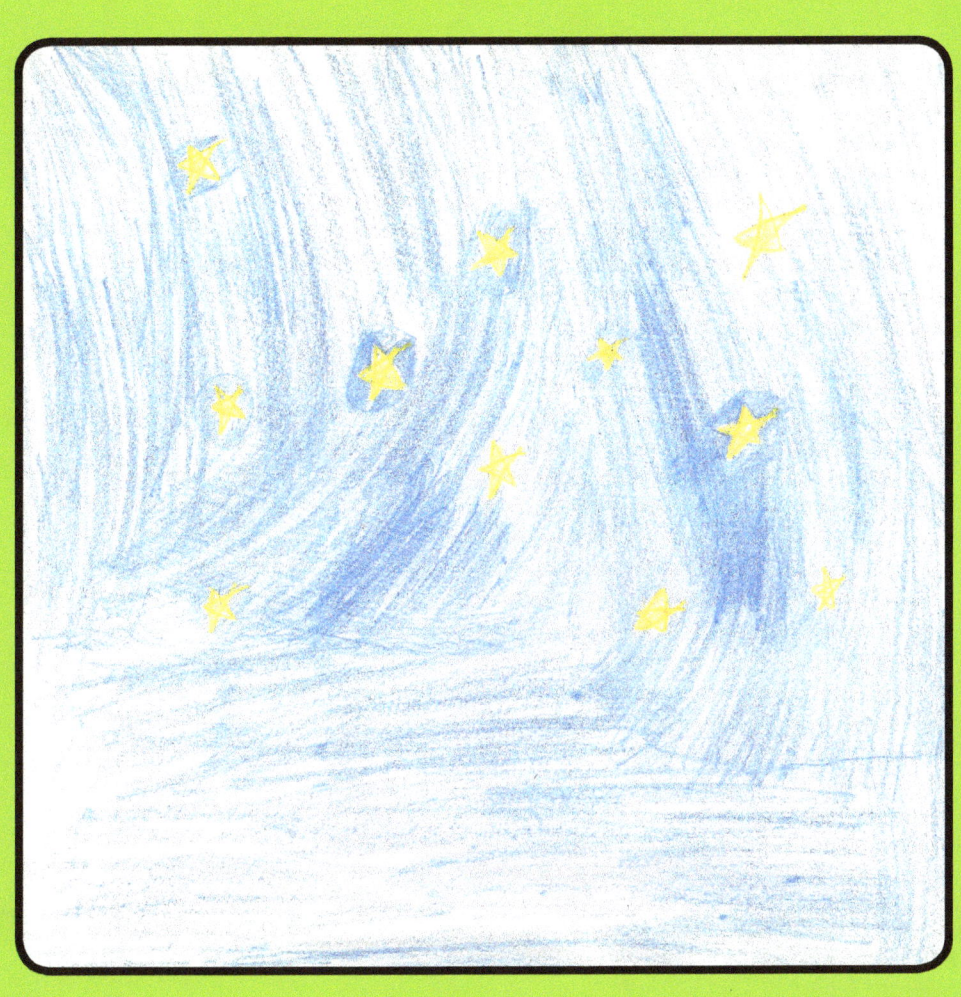

Lord, we thank you for your healing hand.
We thank you for your peace.

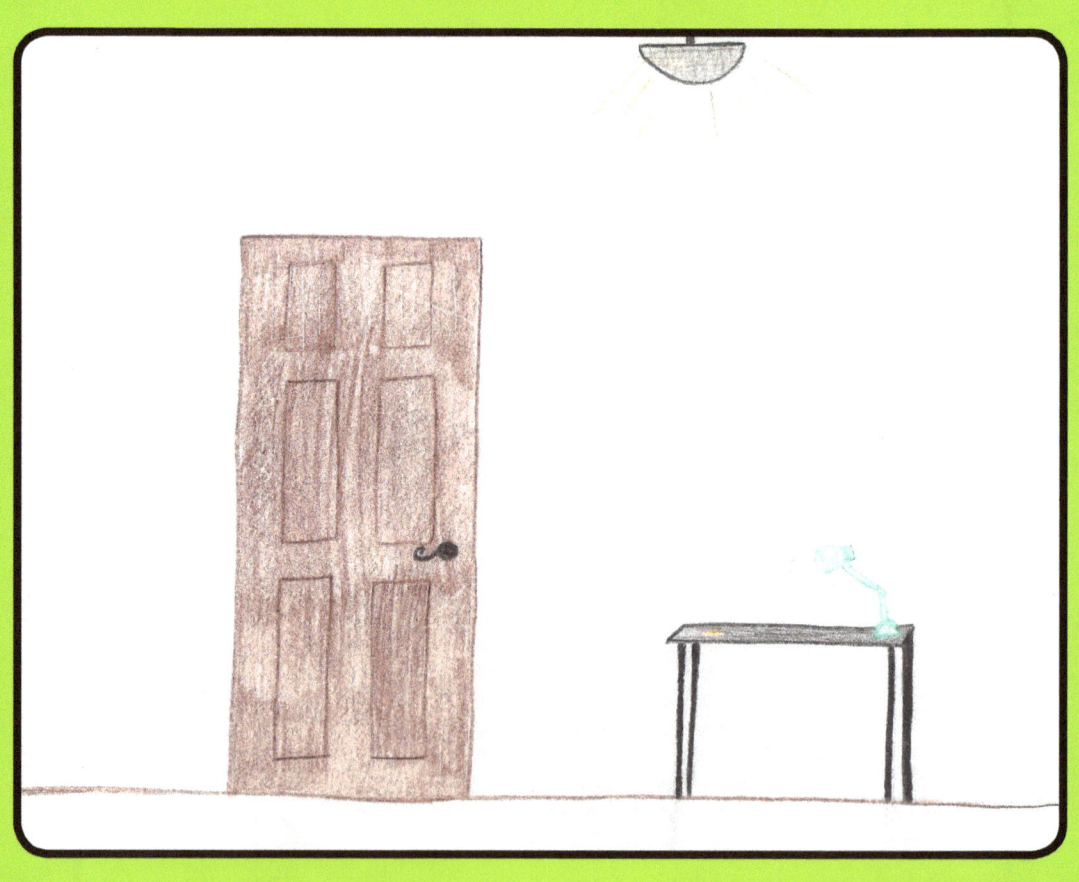

We pray we would fear not

in our fight against this disease.

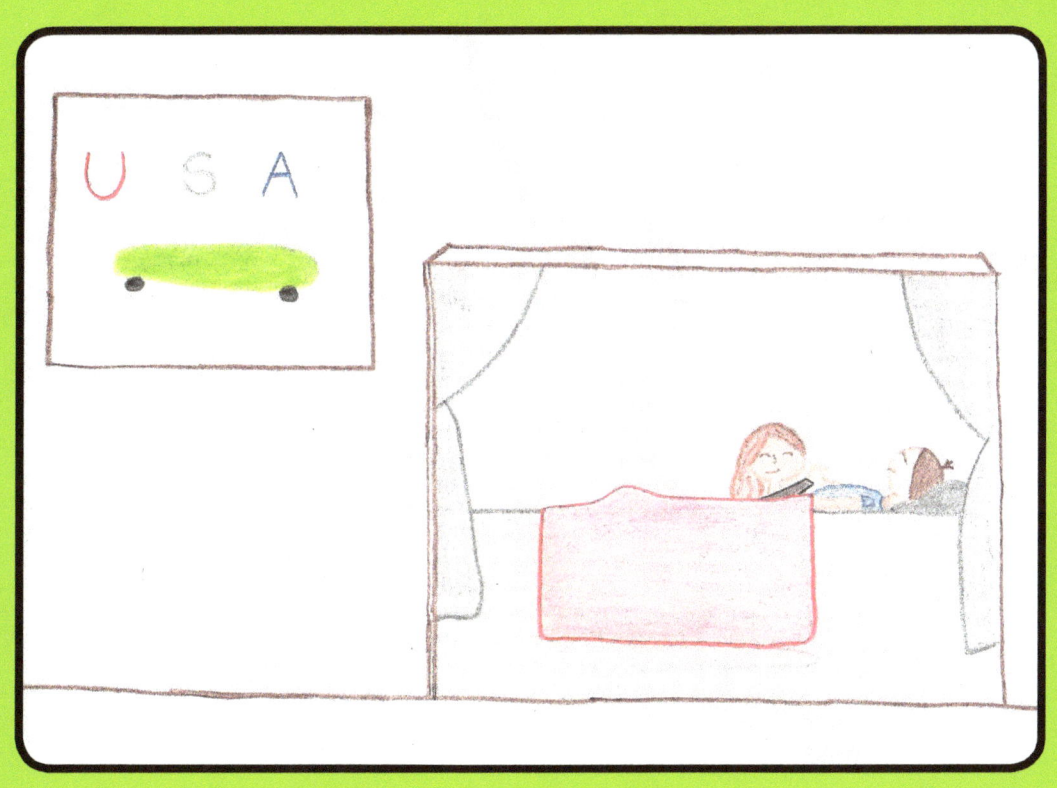

We thank you Lord! We thank you Lord!

We ask your will be done.

We praise your mighty name.

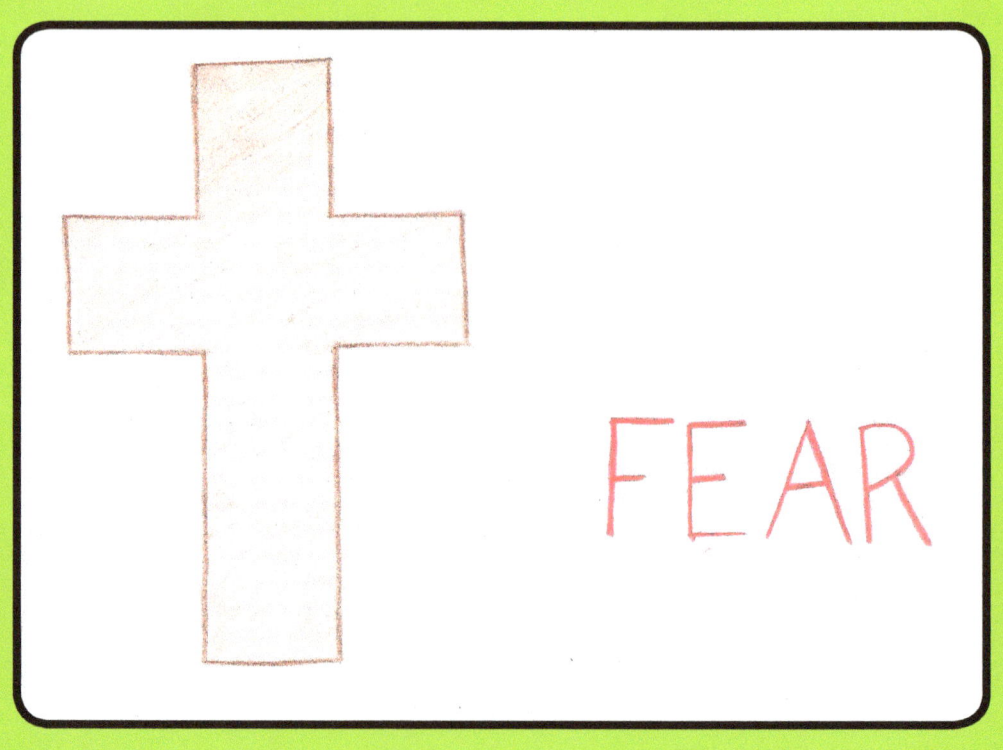

Through you, any battle may be won!
In Jesus name, Amen.

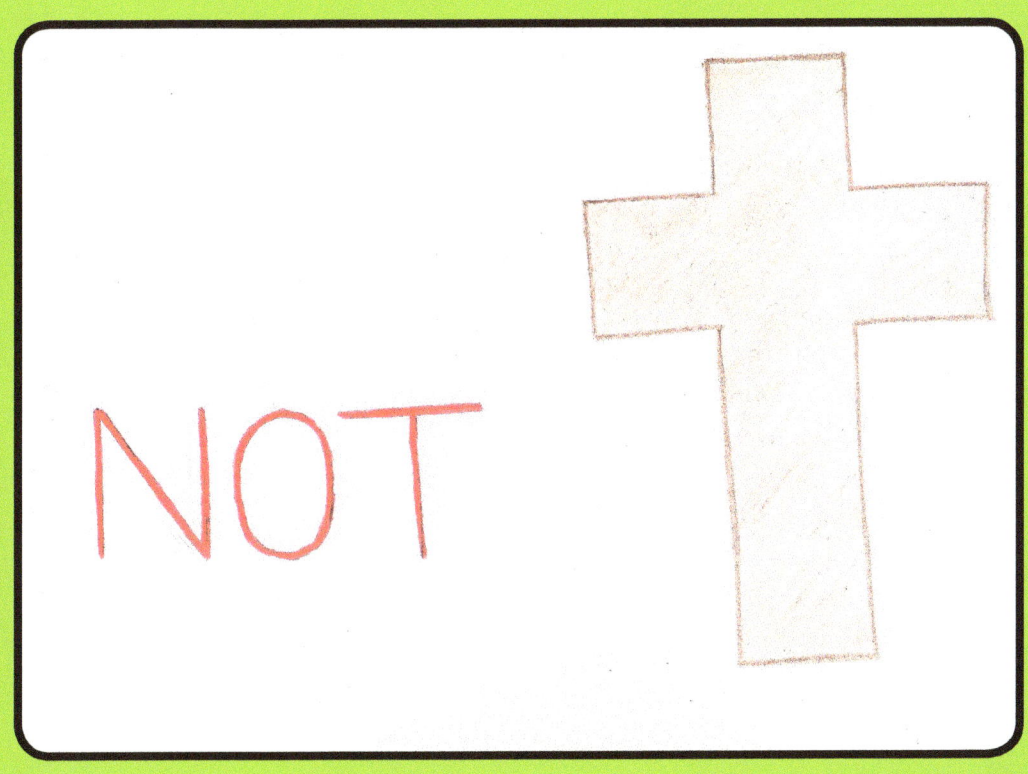

Go to bed my son.

Close your eyes and sleep tight.

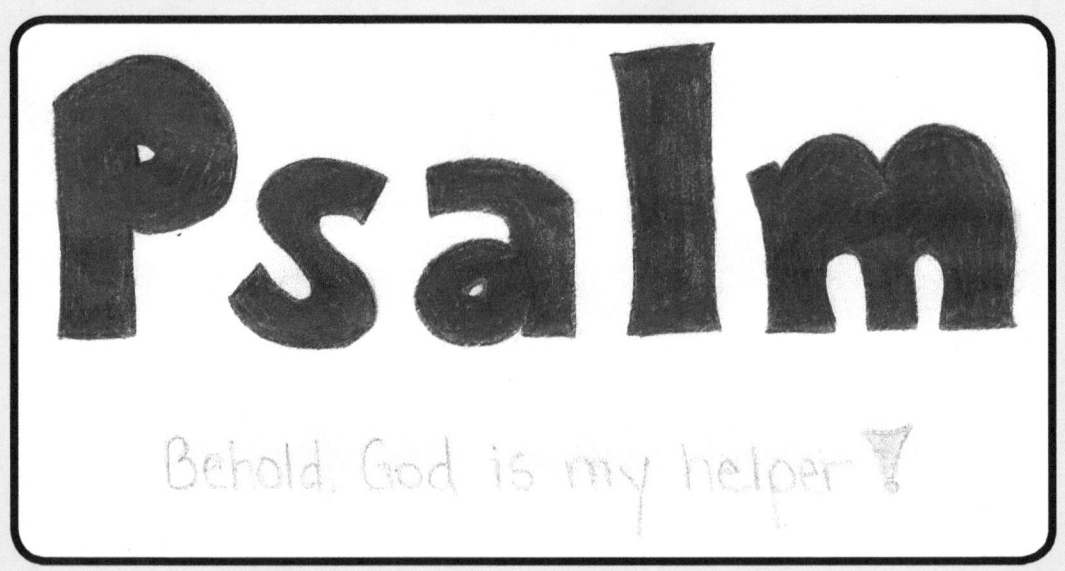

Psalm

Behold, God is my helper!

I love you with all my heart.

I'm so proud of you, goodnight.

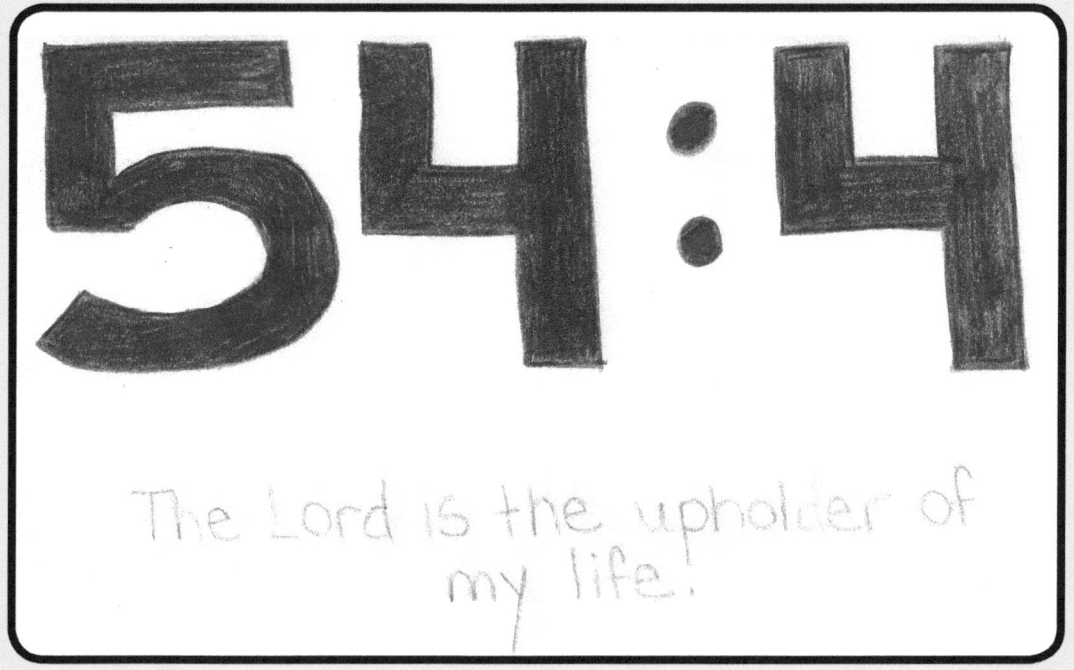

The Lord is the upholder of my life!

WestBow Press books may be ordered through booksellers or by contacting:

WestBow Press
A Division of Thomas Nelson & Zondervan
1663 Liberty Drive
Bloomington, IN 47403
www.westbowpress.com
1 (866) 928-1240

Because of the dynamic nature of the Internet, any web addresses or links contained in
this book may have changed since publication and may no longer be valid. The views
expressed in this work are solely those of the author and do not necessarily reflect the views
of the publisher, and the publisher hereby disclaims any responsibility for them.

Any people depicted in stock imagery provided by Thinkstock are models,
and such images are being used for illustrative purposes only.
Certain stock imagery © Thinkstock.

ISBN: 978-1-5127-4753-9 (sc)
ISBN: 978-1-5127-4754-6 (e)

Library of Congress Control Number: 2016910378

Print information available on the last page.

WestBow Press rev. date: 7/19/2016

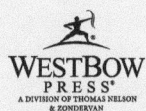

WESTBOW
PRESS®
A DIVISION OF THOMAS NELSON
& ZONDERVAN